# SALICYLATE INTOLERANCE

## and

# THE HEALTHIER I ATE

# THE SICKER I GOT

Revised 2nd Edition 2012

By Joan Tozzi - Ablahani

ISBN 978 - 0 - 615 - 31797- 7

Printed by Lightning Source

I wrote this book about Salicylate Intolerance to help all the people out there suffering from various ailments, being misdiagnosed or being made to think that they are Crazy.

ASPIRIN also known as Acetyl-Salicylic Acid, is the most commonly known Salicylate.[1] It is made from the bark of the Willow tree. Most plants produce Salicylates as a natural insecticide.

I am not a doctor and do not pretend to be one. I do, however, have more personal experience and have researched more information about Salicylate Intolerance than most doctors.

I am one of the lucky ones because I was diagnosed Salicylate Intolerant by an allergy doctor years ago. I was told to avoid Aspirin and wine, period. But he didn't mention fruits, vegetables, Pepto Bismol, Alka Seltzer and the Sodium Salicylate in general anesthesia. However, by knowing that I was intolerant to aspirin, I had something to go on when I hit bottom 2 years ago.

My heart breaks for all the people suffering who don't even know that they are allergic to aspirin. The current generation of children and young adults has never taken aspirin because they have been raised on Tylenol. Therefore, when they suffer from

Asthma, swelling of throat or lips, Arthritis, rashes, ADHD and other symptoms they would never see a connection between their ailments and what they ate yesterday. I pray that they don't suffer for 50 years, like I did, before they discover it can all be prevented.

This book was written in laymen's terms as a starting point since there are no other books written specifically on Salicylate Intolerance. The Medical Field is still in denial about Salicylate Intolerance. Think of all the money the Pharmaceutical Companies would lose if drugs weren't prescribed for migraines, asthma, arthritis, fibromyalgia, hives, dry eyes etc.

I still feel very much alone in my quest to avoid Salicylates and pass the word on to others. There are some excellent web sites where you can further your understanding about Salicylate Intolerance. Without them, I don't know where else I would have turned to for help.

I am living proof that avoiding foods high in Salicylates can prevent those symptoms mentioned and others. God bless you on your Journey. You are not crazy. You are not a hypochondriac. And you are not alone.

I decided to revise my original book about Salicylate Intolerance because in the last 4 years I have researched and learned so much more. While the original book has remained intact I have included much more about sensitivities to artificial colors, artificial flavors, preservatives, fluoride and Gluten Intolerance.

I have included more information about how children's behavior, learning and health are affected by the artificial colors and additives in the food they eat. Hyperactive children should be taken off the chemicals that are affecting them, not put on other drugs. It is my hope that from today on, you will never look at a misbehaving or unfocused child the same way you did in the past.

While my book is not a comprehensive scientific journal, it is an easily understood and well-researched Food Intolerance Handbook written for a layperson to follow while improving their health and quality of life.

I am not vain enough to think that my book is all anyone needs. I generously recommend other helpful websites and books that have helped me. By doing the legwork, and compiling much of the information off the websites, I offer a quick-read informative book that most Doctors will accept more readily than a handful of loose papers copied from the internet.

This book is dedicated to Joe, my loving husband, who patiently put up with my mysterious ailments for 30 years.

# CONTENTS

**MORE ON NEXT PAGE**

# 1 A LIFETIME OF SYMPTOMS

My whole life I was prone to viruses, nausea and dizziness but no fever and surprisingly my sister never caught them. I was either very tired at night or headachy which was a real joy to my wonderful husband of 25 years. As a child, every Sunday after eating spaghetti and meatballs and salad with olive oil and vinegar I would get a headache, so I would take an aspirin. An hour later I would feel worse with a stuffy nose, sore throat, earaches and sometimes vomiting. I missed a lot of school feeling sick very often on Mondays.

When I was 18 years old my allergy doctor told me I was allergic to aspirin which is a Salicylate ( acetyl-salicylic acid ) [1]. That was the reason for the sore throat, stuffy nose ( swelling ) and earaches (swelling and pinching inside ) that I got every Sunday after taking aspirin for my headache.

But what was causing my headaches? I'd have to wait till I was 50 years old and almost died to find out the answer to that mystery. You'll only have to wait one more paragraph. The only thing my allergy Dr. warned me to avoid was aspirin and wine because they are very high in Salicylates.  He forgot to tell me about a hundred other things that are also high in Salicylates.

I experienced many varied symptoms throughout my life which I know now were directly related to eating and drinking Salicylates as well as using toiletries high in Salicylates.

So, what else is high in SALICYLATES ?????????????  (Refer to complete list at end)

I will tell you briefly.  All fruit except bananas and peeled pears, most vegetables except celery, lettuce, string beans, peas, brussel sprouts, beans and cabbage.

Also high are TOMATOS, TOMATO SAUCE, TOMATO PASTE, TOMATO ANYTHING.  TEA, COFFEE, BEER, WINE, VINEGAR, OLIVE OIL, HONEY, ALMONDS, OREGANO, PAPRIKA,

# GINGER, ALLSPICE, CINNAMON, CHILI PEPPER, AND MINTS.[2] All mints, but Wintergreen oil is toxic to someone with a Salicylate Intolerance.[15]

Now that I have your attention I'll continue.     How do you know if you are Salicylate Intolerant? You probably have 2 or more of the following typical symptoms, especially after eating tomato sauce or fruit:

ANGIOEDEMA  - The swelling of something:

Sore throat, swollen salivary glands, swollen eyes,

lips, face, inside of ears, sinuses or stuffy nose.

URTICARIA– Hives, Eczema, or unexplained pink rash on torso.

ASTHMA– Shortness of breath, Look up Sampter Triad on Internet.[4]

ARTHRITIS – achy joints

DRY EYE SYNDROME , Bloodshot eyes

NAUSEA, VERTIGO (dizziness )

MIGRAINES,  headaches (often starting in eyes)

NEUROLOGICAL EFFECTS – hard to focus – Fibro Fog- ADHD

NOSEBLEEDS

Salicylate Intolerance has been linked to ADHD and it's interesting to note that 80% of AUTISTIC children are Salicylate Intolerant. You have to look up Dr. Donna Williams on the internet. She is a Doctor, teacher, writer and artist who was Autistic for 20 years until a very wise Doctor took her off Salicylates . Her story is incredible.

Now let's get back to my lifetime of misdiagnosed Salicylate Intolerance symptoms.  I am qualified to tell you that these symptoms were all directly related to my Salicylate Intolerance. Since avoiding Salicylates they have been significantly reduced.  Please note, that it is almost impossible to completely avoid all Salicylates because they are hidden in everything, especially spices.  Turmeric, MSG, and yellow dye #5 (Tartrazine) which affects many Salicylate Intolerant people are hidden in everything from chips and soups to vitamins.

# 2 BLOODSHOT EYES

For 30 years, I asked my eye Doctor why my eyes were so red. He said my vessels were close to the surface and maybe it was allergies. My eyes always felt gritty and wearing contacts was very difficult. After 20 years I finally gave up. I was told that I had Dry Eye Syndrome and was given Restasis drops. They didn't work at all. I even tried tear duct plugs which were extremely painful and had to be removed 2 days later.

Once I went off Salicylates my eyes cleared up. They are no longer dry and bloodshot. It was one of my reactions to Salicylates. I have actually tested it. When my husband and I went out for dinner recently I put olive oil on my salad and said," watch, my eyes will be beet red tomorrow", and sure enough they were. Just like Dracula. (Italian food is the worst for me with Olive oil, wine, oregano, tomato sauce, basil and balsamic vinegar) By the way you can have Canola Oil, Rice Vinegar and Malt Vinegar.

# 3 HEADACHES

I have had Headaches several times a week my whole life.  Sometimes I would have Migraines, where I would vomit and have to go to bed or just really bad sinus headaches. I know now that they were all Salicylate Intolerant Headaches.  They would always start in my eyes.  This is probably one of my worst symptoms and most constant.  The muscles in my eyes are very affected by my Salicylate Intolerance. They feel weak, sometimes looking back and forth hurts, and my vision gets cloudy.   The Doctors could never figure it out.  Right before I hit bottom and discovered my Salicylate Intolerance I went for a CAT scan because the pain and pressure in my eye was horrible. I thought I had a tumor. The pressure was so bad I thought I had Glaucoma.  I told my Eye Dr. that I wanted to take a pin and pop my eye to relieve the pressure.  OK I am a bit dramatic but it was really bad.   It's all better now.  I can still trigger a headache if I sneak a cup of decaf coffee or eat too much chocolate candy. Yellow dye #5 and high fructose corn syrup seem to give me a headache also and the pain always starts in my right  eye. It's just not worth it, I feel so good without it

# 4 RASHES

Every time I went on vacation south of N.J. I would get a rash from the sun. It ruined my honeymoon and many other vacations in Aruba, Florida, Nevis, Bermuda, Bahamas and even Myrtle Beach. Funny thing was I never used sunscreen in N.J. and never got the rash in N.J.

But I made sure I used sunscreen in tropical sun so I wouldn't burn. Then I would end up with a prickly heat type of rash all over my legs and arms. Guess what's in sunscreen?

OCTYSALATE, HOMOSALATE or other Salicylates. Yes, the rash was from the sunscreen not the sun. Salicylates are absorbed through the skin. In fact, any Menthol such as Ben Gay or Vicks Vaporub is dangerous to anyone who is Salicylate Intolerant. All methyl or menthol containing products are Salicylates. I read an article about a young girl athlete who died from putting too much BenGay on her sore muscles.[15]

There are other skin products that were irritating to me but I didn't know why. Now I do.

I never understood as a teenager why Stridex pads made my acne worse. Stridex and many other acne products are mostly salicylic acid. I always found Acnomel to work very well and it was Sal Free (Salicylate free) . As far as anti – wrinkle facial lotions go, Alpha hydroxy is fine but not Beta hydroxy . Beta is Salicylates. Also, make sure you are not using a hand cream for your dry cracked hands that contains Salicylates. It will only make them worse.

A very dear friend suffered from hives and itchy eczema for many years. She was on several medications for her condition. When she went off Salicylates her skin improved enough to get off most of her medication. It also turns out that the artificial colors in her meds were aggravating the condition more than helping.

And as a final note, don't use common wart or corn remedies. They are all salicylic acid.

# 5 CHAPPED LIPS

My lips were always chapped and burning. The more they burned, the more chapstick or blistex or lipstick I applied. The more chapstick I put on the worse my lips got. I really thought I had acid in my saliva. Well, we all do to some extent to digest our food but I thought I had pure acid. Perhaps the excess salicylic acid that my body couldn't metabolize was in my saliva. Anyway, I didn't know it was a vicious cycle.    Now that I'm using a Sal Free (salicylate free) lipstick, my lips feel fine.   Refer to the lists of Sal Free products on the Guai Support Website.[7] Beware of anything with menthol, aloe or eucalyptus. More recently I discovered that even the artificial colors in Sal Free lipsticks bother me so I have recently switched to an Organic Lipstick called HEMP ORGANICS made with hemp oil and no artificial colors. They feel great.

# 6 MOUTH SORES, CANKER SORES, DRY

# MOUTH

I suffered from mouth sores, canker sores and dry mouth most of my life. While Doctors still don't know exactly what causes canker sores, I suspect that the salicylate acid in Listerine and many other mouth washes may be a culprit. The peppermint, spearmint and wintergreen flavoring in toothpaste is also Salicylates. Beware of wintergreen oil. It is toxic to someone who is Salicylate intolerant.[15] I used Toms of Maine Wintergreen toothpaste once and suffered a very nasty asthma attack. Also, avoid mints and mint gum. You don't have to tell me how difficult this is. I am a teacher and work very closely with my students. Oh well…

All I know is that once I avoided all of the above I stopped getting canker sores and dry mouth. (see page 71 for more information on dry mouth)

So, what do I use? I have recently changed my toothpaste to CLEURE Original Toothpaste, no flavor. ( no mint or menthol ) and I sprinkle BAKING SODA on that to brush my teeth.  Or I use just plain baking soda. Or sometimes I wet my brush, pour a little hydrogen peroxide on my brush then the baking soda on top.  By the way, Baking soda is your friend.  . Since it's an antacid, I'm guessing it helps to get rid of Salicylate ACID as well. This is just a guess.  Sometimes I even take a swig of ½ teaspoon baking soda in a glass of water if I know I've cheated with Salicylates that day.

Since I can't use mints or mouthwash, baking soda helps to freshen my breath by gargling with it and brushing with it.    NO MORE CANKER SORES!!!!!!!!!!!!!!!!

# 7 ARTHRITIS, ACHEY JOINTS

I want to preface this section with a comment about my physical stature. I have always been tall, thin, strong and athletic. That's why all the strange and freaky symptoms I've experienced over the years are so incongruous to an otherwise healthy person. (unless they were in effect being constantly poisoned by food they couldn't metabolize )

During my first pregnancy all my joints over softened and I would frequently just collapse on the floor. At night, if I had to get up to use the bathroom my husband had to carry me because I couldn't walk at all. Since Salicylates cause inflammation in the joints I now wonder if there was a connection. After my 1st son was born I was told that I wasn't immune to Measles and Rubella so they immediately gave me the MMR vaccine. Shortly after, I had achiness in my shoulders, elbows and wrists that lasted for a year. I joined a badminton class with some neighbors but had to quit because I couldn't hold the racket or swing without pain. I assumed my pain was directly related to the vaccine. I now suspect it was a buildup of Salicylates in my system.

After having my second son things went from bad to worse. I could hardly walk for a year (try taking care of 2 kids like this). I mostly crawled or held on to furniture. It felt like someone was putting a knife up my groin and my hip was totally frozen with pain. Of course I still got my normal migraines, nausea, vertigo and achy joints. I was tested for MS, Lyme, Rheumatoid Arthritis and Bone Cancer. (All negative)

I was misdiagnosed with Fibromyalgia and had an exploratory Hernia Operation, which turned out to be totally unnecessary. I was finally diagnosed with OSTEITIS PUBIS, a type of arthritis in the groin area with torn or stretched ligaments and tendons from the pregnancy.

Then I was told that the debilitating pain in my hip was not in any way connected to the Osteitis Pubis. (doctors say this when they have no interest in researching anything unusual)

This was 20 years before the Internet so I marched myself (actually limped) over to the local Hospital Library and looked up Osteitis Pubis. ON MY OWN (again) I found out that the hip adductors are definitely affected when you have Osteitis Pubis and it was all interconnected. Since I knew I was allergic to aspirin and all anti-inflammatory medication, I was given a shot of Cortisone in the groin, which helped.

Was any of this related to my Salicylate Intolerance or was it all the result of carrying a 9 lb.baby? Well, lots of women have 9 lb. babies and don't have all of these joint problems. I believe that if my joints were not in a constant state of inflammation from my Salicylate Intolerance none of these symptoms would have been so severe.

Well life went on and so did my Arthritic symptoms. Arthritis inflammation has a way of finding your most vulnerable spot. Usually an area weakened from an old football injury or in my case an old car accident. At 24 years old I was on my way to work as an Art Teacher and a car ran a stop sign. My whiplash turned into a 30 year chronic stiff neck. I've been going to a chiropractor on and off for 30 years to get periodic relief and physical therapy for the last 3 years. The deep tissue massages and stretching seems to help a little.

However, throughout these 30 years, there have been times when the pain in my lower skull and neck has been so unbearable I wanted to rip my head right off my neck. I'm sure these times with the worst inflammation in my neck and base of my skull were times of very high Salicylate Overload.

# 8 NOSEBLEEDS

My whole life I was very prone to Nosebleeds. My Doctor said that maybe I was lacking in vitamin K which helps with clotting. Of course my sister never had a bloody nose. My parents applied every remedy from rolled up brown paper under the top lip to pinching the bridge of the nose, ice on nose and ice behind the neck. On one occasion, after vomiting a bucket of blood, it was so bad that the Doctor packed my nose with 2 feet of gauze. The next day he removed it and taught me how to make a little pack with rolled tissue. It was ingenious. I have helped hundreds of friends and strangers by making a pack to stop their nosebleeds. It's so simple yet so effective.

Now, the million-dollar question. Why did I get so many nosebleeds? Well, if Salicylates were causing inflammation in the vessels of my bloodshot eyes, why not in my nose too. Since avoiding foods high in Salicylates the nosebleeds are gone.

# 9 THE YEAR THE LIGHT BULB WENT ON

In November 2006 my son, a senior in high school was playing Varsity Football. He came down with a very bad case of Mononucleosis. It went into Hepatitis, which means his liver was inflamed, as well as his spleen. His symptoms were high fever, sore throat, swollen glands, vomiting, coughing and achiness. It was at my insistence that they even tested him for Mono since his symptoms were atypical. Some kids just get a mild case with low fever, mild sore throat and fatigue; many totally unaware that they even have it.

After a month of caring for my son, night and day, coming home lunchtime from work to give him his pills and force him to eat and drink, I became very stressed out and run down.

AND THE HEALTHIER I ATE THE SICKER I GOT. Hey, I was putting apple cider vinegar in my water every day because I read that it was good for Arthritis. I was putting cranberries on my high fiber cereal. I was eating almonds and having a V-8 juice every day. I was drinking 5 cups of green tea everyday with honey in it. How healthy can you get?  I was eating lots of fruits and vegetables, making homemade grapefruit juice and putting olive oil and vinegar on my salad.

## I WAS KILLING MYSELF !!!!!!!!!!!!

My son started with the Mono in November 2006.  I started with Arthritis like achiness in every joint in my body in December 2006 and had swollen glands. (Like I get from aspirin)

I went for blood work to rule out Mono and Lyme disease.  I was given an antibiotic for the swollen glands. (And of course I took my probiotic acidophilus to replace the good bacteria that antibiotics kill)

When the swollen glands didn't go away I was given a $2^{nd}$ dose of antibiotics.  Meanwhile I kept eating all my healthy foods and even started making homemade grapefruit juice by boiling cut-up sections of grapefruit with the skin on.  I read this helped to boost your immune system.

## OH, I WAS BOOSTING SOMETHING ALL RIGHT, MY SALICYLATE OVERLOAD!!!!!!!!!!!!!!!!!!!!!!!!!!

By January 2007 I had achy joints, swollen glands and then my Asthma kicked in real bad so I went to my Allergy/Asthma doctor.  Also in January I had packed up our shore house and stored most of it in a friend's basement, which smelled very moldy. If you are sensitive to mold and mildew you can smell it immediately. I am. I can.

I told my asthma doctor that my asthma was probably a very bad reaction to my exposure to mold. It made sense and she put me on Prednisone and told me to use the Nebulizer with Pulmicort and Albuterol 3X's a day. I continued to get worse and worse. I was so short of breath I could hardly breathe. I continued to go to work as an Art Teacher but could barely talk to my students because of the severe asthma. I called my doctor after 3 weeks and told her that nothing was working and that I was still very short of breath. She told me to just continue using the Nebulizer, which actually made me feel worse. I thought that maybe I had a blockage so I went to my cardiologist. Everything was fine in that department.

After a month of Asthma and shortness of breath I woke up one morning crying and I said to my husband, " I FEEL LIKE I'M GOING TO DIE AND MY DOCTORS ARE GOING TO LET ME DIE.''

"I guess it's all up to me to cure myself. Let me think, what am I allergic to? ASPIRIN! "

Gee, Aspirin (Salicylates ) gives me a sore throat, swollen glands, stuffy nose and makes the inside of my ears pinch. At this point, that's all I had to go on. I didn't realize all the other symptoms that Salicylates were responsible for.

I wondered if there were Salicylates in any foods. So I went on the Internet and typed in 'FOODS CONTAINING SALICYLATES '.

To my horror, I discovered all fruits are high in Salicylates except bananas and peeled pears. Most vegetables except string beans, peas, celery, lettuce, beans, cabbage and brussel sprouts.

Others that are very high are wine, beer, tea, coffee, all vinegar (except malt and rice, ) honey, mints, almonds, tomato paste, tomato sauce, mushrooms, cucumbers and broccoli. Salicylates are extremely high (and the hardest to avoid) in spices like oregano, basil, rosemary, thyme, ginger, paprika , chili pepper ( forget buffalo wings ) yellow dye #5 and turmeric . And believe it or not, OLIVE OIL is extremely high, but you can have CANOLA OIL, which is just as good for your heart.[12, 13, 14]

You don't get an immediate effect after eating these foods high in Salicylates, as you would from a food allergy because a Food Intolerance is cumulative. It's the BUCKET

THEORY.  When the bucket is full from eating too many Salicylates you can have a full-blown attack.

Struggling to breathe, I sat at my computer, mesmerized, reading everything I could about Salicylate Intolerance. What I read brought tears to my eyes.  I WAS NOT ALONE. Here were all the true accounts of other people suffering their whole lives until they discovered the truth about Salicylate Intolerance.

My heart broke for the little girl who felt sick all the time especially every Sunday after spaghetti dinner (me).

# GET READY TO RUMBLE

Now, I was on a mission to get better.  I stopped the nebulizer and all the medication that actually made me feel sicker.  Although the list of foods to avoid was extensive, I stopped eating everything containing Salicylates.  Two days after avoiding these foods I started getting better.

# 2 DAYS AFTER AVOIDING THESE FOODS I GOT BETTER !!!!

I want to shout it from the rooftops.  That's why I wrote this book.

Let me say this again: *Two days after avoiding these foods high in Salicylates I started getting better:*

1) By the end of the week my breathing improved 100%

2) My achiness in all my joints was gone.

3) My bloodshot eyes and dry eyes cleared up.

4) My headaches were gone.

5) My swollen glands got better.

6) My occasional bloody noses are gone.

7) My constipation and hemorrhoids are better.

8)  And I have more energy.

All of these symptoms can and do return if I cheat or unknowingly eat foods containing Salicylates.

Two weeks after cutting out Salicylates from my diet I made copies of the information that I got off the Internet and went to visit my Allergy/Asthma Doctor and my Family Doctor. I told them that I was all better. I said, "You know I'm allergic to aspirin, it's in my file, but did you know that Salicylates are also in all the foods on this list. I was eating all the ones in the extremely high column. When I stopped eating all Salicylates I got all better in a week."

My Asthma/Allergy Doctor said," OK, that makes sense." My Family Doctor, who is a vegetarian, was in complete denial. He said, "No, that can't be true. Fruits and vegetables are good for you. The Salicylates in food must be different from the ones in aspirin." He was dead wrong. The only difference is the amount. Eat enough fruit and it will add up to the same amount of Salicylates in an aspirin.

The reason I probably ate so many foods high in Salicylates and became hypersensitive to them was because I have read Prevention Magazine for 30 years. It was my health bible. If they said to eat blueberries, I ate blueberries and almonds and olive oil and cranberries and apple cider vinegar and cinnamon and green tea etc. Never once did they say, "Caution limit intake if allergic to aspirin." Which I feel would have been the responsible thing to do.

Don't get me wrong, a majority of the population should eat Salicylates. It's a natural anti-inflammatory. However, it causes inflammation and is poison to those of us who are Salicylate Intolerant. In high enough doses it is actually toxic to everyone but we all have our own tolerance level. Mine happens to be very low.

# 10 SALICYLATES AND ASTHMA EPIDEMIC

Unbeknownst to most people, scientists have genetically altered fruits and vegetables to produce more Salicylates[16]. Since it is a plant's natural insecticide, it discourages the pests from eating them. The more natural Salicylates a plant produces, the less pesticide a farmer needs to use, which is better for the environment.

However, this has backfired. There is now a higher concentration of Salicylates in all of our fruits and vegetables including those that are processed into baby food. Little babies cannot ingest as much Salicylates as adults without some adverse effects such as rashes, hives, swelling on face, Asthma and other breathing problems. High Salicylates have also been linked to ADHD and AUTISM.[8]

# 11 ADHD and AUTISM

Over the past 2 years I have read and researched so much about Salicylate Intolerance that most of it has become imbedded in my brain as general knowledge. I wrote most of this book off the top of my head, even forgetting where some of my information originally came from.

I have read that ADHD in children can be greatly improved by avoiding Salicylates, artificial flavorings, food dyes and preservatives such as MSG, Sodium Nitrate, Yellow Dye #5, Tartrazine and Benzoates.

If you have a child with ADHD you would be wise to check out the FEINGOLD DIET and website as well as the FAILSAFE DIET and website.[5]

I have also read that 80% of Autistic children are Salicylate Intolerant.[5] This connection makes me want to jump up for joy that maybe these children can be helped, but it also makes me want to cry that they aren't being told about the connection.

You must look up Dr. Donna Williams and read about her whole life experience being Autistic, being taken off Salicylates and other food chemicals by a very wise doctor and going on to become a Doctor, a Writer, a Teacher and an Artist.[5, 6]

I know that Salicylates have a profound neurological effect on people who are Salicylate Intolerant. You feel foggy headed and it becomes difficult to concentrate. (often called Fibro Fog ) I know, I was a chronic day dreamer. Somehow, I was able to compensate and get very good grades, ( I graduated with Honors ) but it took me a long time to do homework and I needed total silence, no distractions. I don't know how kids do homework in front of the TV.

It's possible that Autistic children cannot tolerate any level of Salicylates in food or any food chemicals like preservatives, artificial flavorings and artificial colorings. You know, Autistic children aren't born with Autistic behavior. Something triggers it. I just know how I feel when I get that foggy headed feeling, when the Salicylates go right to my brain and I can't think straight. The greatest teacher in the world would not be able to penetrate that fog to teach me anything when I feel like that. Again, I am not a doctor and I am simply musing over things that I have read.

The FEINGOLD DIET and the FAILSAFE DIET present a sounder argument than I could ever summarize here. I HOPE THIS INSPIRES YOU TO DO YOUR OWN RESEARCH.

# 12 FIBROMYALGIA

I already mentioned that years ago I was misdiagnosed with Fibromyalgia. I would get migraines, nausea, vertigo, every joint in my body ached and I had chronic fatigue. At 40 I started getting Asthma. I have proven to myself that these same symptoms can be prevented by avoiding Salicylates. However, most doctors are taught that all these symptoms add up to Fibromyalgia. They are not sure what causes it and there's no cure. So they treat the symptoms.

There is a wonderful website for people with Fibromyalgia called Guai Support that lists everything containing Salicylates. You can look up everything such as food products, cosmetics, toiletries, shampoos, hand lotions, cleansers and medications.

One of the treatments for Fibromyalgia is Guaifenesin. It is one of the main ingredients in Cough Medicine which thins mucous. Several studies have shown that Salicylates block the effects of Guaifenesin. So the Guai Support website lists everything containing Salicylates for people with Fibromyalgia to avoid.

This list is a God-send for everyone who is Salicylate Intolerant. Now try to follow my thinking here. All the people with Fibromyalgia are prescribed Guaifenesin, but are told to avoid all Salicylates because it blocks the effect of Guaifenesin. Suddenly all of their symptoms, headaches, achiness, arthritis, fatigue, dizziness, nausea, and Fibro Fog disappear. Well it seems to me that the Guaifenesin has less to do with their recovery than the avoidance of all Salicylates.

I am inclined to believe that eventually the Medical Field will have to acknowledge the fact that Fibromyalgia was a catch all diagnosis for a cluster of symptoms associated with Salicylate Intolerance. My misdiagnosis of Fibromyalgia was indeed Salicylate Intolerance and my symptoms are now gone.

# 13 NURSING BABIES AND SALICYLATE

# INTOLERANCE

I nursed my first son. He was the Colicky one. Both my sons were extreme spitter-uppers, 20 times a day, a puddle of spit up on the floor, on the couch or on my shirt. I didn't nurse my second son and he was extremely happy and never cried.

My first son, Mr. Colicky, cried all the time, sometimes for hours on end. They say that if a Mom is Salicylate Intolerant and eats a lot of Salicylates the unmetabolized Salicylates are passed on to the baby through the breast milk .[8] This is not good since babies can't tolerate more than a very small amount.

I nursed my son for 3 months. My son was colicky for exactly 3 months. Then he turned into a sweet happy baby. He was fine the next 3 months on formula. There's no such thing as coincidence. When I started feeding him baby food at 6 months he started getting strange circular rashes. They would start out like a red outline of a circle which would eventually fill in solid red. My Doctor didn't know they were hives. Back then didn't either.  My Doctor actually said that he thought it was an imprint from my son's button on his shirt.   Ten buttons scattered all over his chest???!!!

These rashes occurred at the same time I started feeding my son baby food sweet potatoes, spinach, squash, applesauce, beets, peaches and plums, all high in Salicylates.

As my son got older, he was able to tell me that all fruit, (except bananas) made his throat itch.  At the time I didn't know about Salicylate Intolerance so I didn't believe him. I made him eat some fruit.  We also had spaghetti sauce several days a week, macaroni and broccoli drank a lot of iced tea and apple juice. No wonder my kids were so hyper.

(See chapter 17 which explains how some babies are very sensitive to the Corn Syrup in Formula )

# 14 FLUORIDE AND SALICYLATE

# INTOLERANCE

Fluoride which has always been heralded as the great tooth decay preventer is also sold as rat poison.5 But weren't we all told to give our babies fluoride drops every week to prevent cavities? Thank God I always forgot to.

It turns out that Fluoride actually increases the adverse effect of Salicylates in Salicylate Intolerant people. Eating toothpaste can cause fluoride toxicity, which can actually kill a child, cause fluorosis of the bones or at least cause gastro intestinal inflammation. It can lower your IQ and increase your chance of getting Alzheimer's.

Fluoride is only effective in preventing cavities if applied topically on the teeth then rinsed off without swallowing any of it. (and even that is now being challenged) It was never intended to be taken orally. Putting it in our drinking water is short of slow acting genocide. If you Google the dangers of fluoride you will even see an article that explains how the Nazis put fluoride in the drinking water to dummy-down the masses and make people more docile. 22

Companies producing Aluminum products and Phosphate Fertilizers end up with fluoride as a toxic waste. It is very expensive and difficult to dispose of. Back in the 1950's someone came up with the insane idea and persuaded the FDA and our government to buy the poison at a 20,000% markup and put it into our drinking water.

Today 99% of western Europe has banned fluoridation. Only 5% of the world is still subjected to fluoride in their water with 50% living in North America.[23]

You must see the full-length documentary from Australia called FIRE WATER. It is produced by Sapphire Eyes Docos and can be seen on You Tube at www.youtube.com/watch?v=6SMKemanUQ8 . It is about Australia's Industrial Fluoridation Disgrace and how the people are fighting it. It is incredible.

Does it even surprise you that I ate toothpaste as a kid? Of course my mother never knew. My girlfriend and I would squeeze toothpaste along the top of a glass of water and have a toothpaste cocktail. That, in combination with my already high in Salicylates Italian Diet would make for one very sick little girl. I'm sure that night I would have one of my many stomachaches, headaches and perhaps dizziness and vomiting. " OH NO, JOAN HAS ANOTHER VIRUS."

# 15 GENERAL ANESTHESIA AND

# SALICYLATE INTOLERANCE

I always had a severe reaction to general anesthesia. Now I know the reason. There is Sodium Salicylate in most anesthesia to address the pain and inflammation during surgery. However, if you are Salicylate Intolerant, they are literally pumping you up with poison.

A friend of mine told me that his lips swell when he eats Tomato Sauce. He knows he's allergic to aspirin and he has very bad Asthma. Last year he had minor surgery and stopped breathing during surgery. I'm sure it was from the Sodium Salicylate.

Even when an Aspirin Allergy Alert is in someone's' file, the doctors still don't connect the dots from Salicylic Acid (aspirin) to Sodium Salicylate in anesthesia. THIS DUMBFOUNDS ME. Some people do die during surgery while under general anesthesia. I believe a lot of these people were Salicylate Intolerant and didn't know it.

Many people are also allergic to the preservative in anesthesia called Sodium Metabisulfite.

At 18 I had 4 impacted wisdom teeth removed in the hospital. The whole day, as relatives came to visit, my Mom would say, "Joan, your sister is here," but I couldn't seeEverything was like a kaleidoscope. And when I tried to look up I would throw up. This went on all day. When you are Salicylate Intolerant waking up from anesthesia is so scary. You can hear everyone but you can't see or focus. You can't talk well to communicate but you know you are going to throw up all the poison pumped into you. The Salicylates have a major effect on your brain and eye muscles. Since I had several minor surgeries in my twenties, I experienced this several times.

At 35 my husband brought me to the hospital early in the morning for Same Day Surgery. At 3:00 pm I remember a nurse saying to my husband, "We have to wake her up," then she starting smacking my face saying "Mrs. Ablahani you have to wake up now." She told my husband to get on one side of me and help walk me. I couldn't see clearly because my eyes wouldn't open more than a slit. I was able to say, "I'm gonna throw up," and I did. At 7:00 pm they had to admit me overnight because I couldn't stop throwing up. They had given me anti nausea needles 3 times but that doesn't remove the toxic overload of Salicylates from your body. I guess the vomiting helps. By 9:00pm I stopped vomiting from the Same Day Surgery and I felt better.

At 36 years old I needed a Hernia Operation. I told the Surgeon that I have a severe reaction to General Anesthesia and could I have the operation with Local Anesthesia. Hesaid he never did it before with just local but we could try. The operation was fine, I was awake but sedated and I felt wonderful when it was over.

Back then, I had no idea that there were Salicylates in General Anesthesia. Now I actually wear a Medical Alert Bracelet stating that I am Salicylate Intolerant including Sodium Salicylate in Anesthesia. If I am in a car accident and unconscious I don't want the doctors to poison me with Salicylates on top of it.

# 16 GINGER AND MOTION SICKNESS

Whenever we were sick and nauseous my mother gave us Ginger Ale. It was common knowledge that ginger helped nausea and motion sickness. Because I was prone to motion sickness I would take Ginger Capsules every time I traveled with my husband and kids. Every time we reached our destination, my husband and the boys would go to the pool while Mommy would be sick and have to lie down for a few hours. And you wonder why they call me the Fun Vacuum. Needless to say, the last time we flew to Florida I didn't take anything and I felt fine. Ginger is extremely high in Salicylates and was causing me to be sick.

# 17 DR. DORIS RAPP – THE DONAHUE SHOW

In 1988 the Donahue Show featured The Mother of Environmental Medicine, Dr.Doris Rapp. I saw the video 2 years ago and it was a real eye opener. She wrote the book, "Is This Your Child?" and many other good books about how food, chemicals and other toxins in the environment affect our health and behavior.

She discovered the Provocation/Neutralization method of treating allergies. The video shows actual children who are given 1 pea or 1 drop of what they are allergic to. (provocation). Then you see some of them become aggressive, punching and kicking or laughing like they're drunk, or crawling under a table depressed or crying or just spaced out and unfocused.

Several minutes later they were injected with a very diluted serum of what they are sensitive to. (neutralization). They immediately returned to happy, quiet, seemingly well adjusted children. Seeing this was enough to convince me that all of the children in my class that are hyperactive, misbehaving or totally spaced out and unfocused are being affected by something.

More effort should be made to find out what they are sensitive to before arbitrarily putting them on Ritalin, Adderall or other drugs. It just makes more sense to remove what's affecting them, not camaflouging the symptoms with a zombie creating, mind altering drug.

I have seen students who are fine before lunch become off the wall, calling out and interrupting me after lunch. Close examination shows that they were affected by artificially colored and flavored slushee drinks, pizza, ketchup, doritos or cheese doodles with yellow#5, jolly ranchers or other colored candy.

One extremely hyperactive boy told me that he ate Froot Loops for breakfast every day. He took my advise to have eggs or a plain cereal like cherrios. (the organic ones with no BHT is better) The next day he came in calmer and said he felt more clear headed. He actually felt a difference and it showed in his behavior. Another little boy whose mother read my book decided to avoid everything with yellow dye #5. He said he felt more focused and it showed.

The following is a list of actual children in my class who were not ready to make a dietary change: Some had the same symptoms that I got rid of by going low Sal.

- A girls with Juvenile Arthritis on medication

- A girl with red dry eyes. She tried plugs than had surgery on tear ducts.

- A boy with ADHD and Bi-polar disorder.

- A boy with ADHD and ODD

- A boy with Tourette Syndrome

- And the kids with headaches, nosebleeds, , achy joints, eczema and asthma

Here are a few of the typical symptoms to alert you that your INFANT may have Food Intolerances or allergies: (complete list in book, "Is This Your Child?") Colic, Excessive spitting-up, Vomiting, Diarrhea/Constipation, Nose/Chest congestion, Eczema, Rashes, Screaming, Prolonged crying, Dislike of cuddling, Excessive drooling, Extreme perspiration, Crib rocking, Head banging, Early walking 7-10 months, Ear infections, Removes clothing,

Some symptoms of possible Allergy in TODDLERS: Red earlobes, Red cheeks, Dark eye circles, Bags under eyes, Wrinkles under eyes, Spaced out look, Wiggly legs, Dislike of being touched or cuddled, Recurrent infections of Ears, Chest or Sinuses, Coughing, Wheezing, Bloating, Gas, Vomiting, Headaches,

Nose Rubbing, Temper tantrums, Clinging, Whining, Hyperactivity,

Aggression ( Biting, Hitting, Kicking)

My niece's 2-month-old baby boy had severe colic. They had already

switched his formula to Soy because it seemed he was in very bad

gastrointestinal stress. He would scream and cry before eating and after

eating. She slept over one night and after witnessing that poor baby in pain I

took a look at her formula. Did you realize that CORN SYRUP is in most Baby

Formulas ? Regular and Soy ? I went to the Pharmacy and couldn't find one

without corn syrup. MANY BABIES AND ADULTS ARE ALLERGIC TO CORN.

Corn is a GMO (genetically modified organism) modified to be able to

tolerate higher levels of pesticides.) Then Corn Syrup is made by processing

Corn Starch with many chemicals. It has become commonly accepted that

corn syrup is bad for everyone so WHAT IS IT DOING IN BABY FORMULA

???????????????

That night I ordered an organic Soy Formula made with Brown Rice Syrup

called Baby's Only on the internet. I gave it to my niece and 2 days later she

called to say , "Thank You So Much. He is officially a new happy baby."

# 18 RACHEL CARSON – ENVIRONMENTAL SCIENCE

As a young girl in the late 1960's I played outside everyday, climbing trees, climbing down the red shale cliff that led to the brook (Peter's Brook) behind our house and playing in the ravine next to our house. I loved nature. I would catch minnows, crayfish and tadpoles and find toads, snakes and salamanders under rocks. Then gradually I saw less and less of living creatures in and around the brook.

Now that I've read about Rachel Carson, a lot of this makes sense. She was an American Marine Biologist in the 1960's and a Pioneer in Environmental Science. At that time a lot of Chemical companies were making a lot of money producing about 1000 new chemicals with no regard for long term effects. They would spray DDT haphazardly over communities to kill mosquitos and beetles. During WW II it did help in fighting Typhoid and Malaria but at what cost.

Bugs can mutate faster than other wildlife and it turned out that DDT was more deadly to birds, the environment and human health.

In 1962 Rachel Carson wrote a book called "Silent Spring" questioning the logic of using chemicals that have such a bad effect on the environment. (DDT was responsible for the threat of extinction of the Bald Eagle). She said the DDT was ending up in our soil, in the worms which the birds ate, in the plants that humans ate and eventually in our bones.

Her book caused such an uproar that President Kennedy had a Scientific Advisory committee look into it and that prompted the birth of the EPA (Environmental Protection Agency) and the eventual ban of DDT.

I'm sure now that the disappearance of fish and other marine life in Peter's Brook was directly related to the spraying of DDT in our town as well as the dumping of other chemical pollutants in the rivers before it also was eventually banned.

I sadly ponder if maybe my playing in the brook as a child didn't somehow contribute to my MCS. (multiple chemical sensitivities)

# 19 FEINGOLD AND FAILSAFE DIETS

At about the same time in the 1960's that Rachel Carson was discovering how bad DDT and other chemicals were for the environment, Dr. Ben Feingold started noticing an increase in behavior problems, learning problems, ADHD, asthma and chronic ear infections. His tests showed that certain synthetic food additives (colors, flavors, preservatives and artificial sweeteners) had an adverse effect on learning, behavior and overall health in sensitive people.

Dr. Feingold was treating several newlywed women for asthma. None of them had a previous history of asthma. It was eventually traced back to the artificial colors in their birth control pills.

So many children (including my own) become sicker while taking liquid medicine or pills for cough, infections, fever or runny noses because of the artificial colors (red, pink, purple, yellow, orange, green) sweeteners (aspartame, splenda) and artificial flavors (cherry, grape, bubblegum ). It is unconscionable to think that the little people who are the most affected by these additives have the most added into their medicine.

My son used to vomit for days, hallucinate, have night terrors and high fevers probably started by his food intolerances and then intensified by the artificial colors and flavors.

THE FEINGOLD DIET (Feingold.org) eliminates:

-ALL ARTIFICIAL COLORS – YELLOW DYE #5 ( Tartrazine ) also called E-102 is possibly the worst. Made from coal tar, it is an Industrial Waste Product used to color food, cosmetics and other products. It can cause Migraines, Asthma, ADD, ADHD, OCD, ODD, Thyroid Cancer , Lupus, Eczema, Hives ,Angioedema (swelling). Other artificial colors all made from Petroleum - YELLOW DYE# 6, RED 3, RED 40, BLUE 1 , BLUE 2, GREEN 3 and ORANGE B. A group of synthetic dyes to also avoid are the AZO dyes including Amaranth.

-PRESERVATIVES – BHA, BHT, TBHQ, Nitrates, Benzoates, and Sulfites.

-ARTIFICIAL FLAVORS and FLAVOR ENHANCERS - Most artificial flavors are a combination of many chemicals. Artificial coffee flavor is as many as 100 different chemicals. Vanillin (artificial vanilla) is the industrial waste product of Paper Mills. Some things are added to enhance flavors like MSG.

-Natural Salicylates in Foods. (see lists of foods in back of book)

The FAILSAFE DIET ([www.fedup.com.au](www.fedup.com.au) ) was devised by Anne Swain  a

dietician in conjunction with other allergists affiliated with the RPAH (Royal

Prince Alfred Hospital ) in Australia. It has been around since the 1980's and

eliminates all of the above as well as chemicals and salicylates in the

environment that we inhale such as household cleaners, pesticides, toiletries and

perfumes. [19]

The Failsafe Diet also encourages you to use the ELIMINATION DIET  to test

further for a sensitivity to  Salicylates, Amines, Glutamates and Oxylates.

 Salicylates are a chemical occurring naturally in food as a pesticide and is

highest in unripened fruits and vegetables. They tend to decrease as food ripens.

Amines are a chemical that increases as foods age and ferment. Foods like meat,

fish, cheese, wine, bananas and chocolate.  Some people become violently ill from

amines and need to eat extremely fresh meat and fish and avoid aged cheeses,

wine and chocolate.

The ELIMINATION DIET  is a good way to figure out what you are sensitive to.

(Always do under a Doctors care ) By eliminating all foods except chicken, rice

and water and then adding things back in one at a time you are able to see what you react to.  I didn't do it because I already knew that I was allergic to aspirin.

So I cut out the Salicylates in the moderate to very high column and in 2 days I

was cured of Asthma, Arthritis, Migraines, Dizziness, Vomiting, Nosebleeds,

Swollen Saliva Glands, Red Dry Eyes and a Foggy Headed Feeling.  Some other

less severe symptoms persisted so I eventually had to avoid  Gluten and Dairy.

While the Elimination Diet is good for some people it can cause withdrawal

symptoms (which I didn't experience by just cutting out moderate to very high

sals) and then other severe symptoms when first starting to add foods back in,

even foods low in salicylates.  When we completely remove an allergy trigger we

can become hypersensitive to it when re-exposed to it. That's why I recommend

cutting out all of the high and very high salicylates, most of the moderates, but

continue eating the foods that are low in sals.

The information I've obtained from the Feingold Association and Fedup.com.au

is probably the main reason I decided to update my book.  I recommend that

everyone view the Symptoms and Success Stories on  Feingold.org  I am

continually encouraged and able to help other people with the up to date

information I have found in the Feingold Pure Facts Newsletter.

By avoiding Artificial Colors, Flavors, Additives, Preservatives and Salicylates Feingold Members claim to have been cured or have seen a great improvement in the following symptoms:(as well as the ones in the complete list in the back) Autism 23 and many symptoms on the Autistic Spectrum, ADD, ADHD, Asperger, OCD, ODD, Asthma, Acid Reflux, Bipolar disorder, Hives, Swelling, Migraines, Ear Infections, Tinnitus, Epilepsy, Tourette's and Eczema.

It is interesting to note that most people with a Food or Chemical Intolerance have a short fuse, are impatient or easily upset. Since I have gotten off most Salicylates, artificial colors and other chemical toxins, I am calmer and more patient.

# 20  BANNING ARTIFICIAL FOOD DYES

I referenced much of this information on the History of Food Coloring from the book "Why Your Child is Hyperactive" by Ben F. Feingold, MD

Before Abe Lincoln there was no formal Food Industry in the U.S. People used natural colors and preserved their food with spices, smoke and salt. In 1865, after the Civil War, the development of cities necessitated new means of processing food. There were no regulations yet and many of the preservatives and colors were toxic. Formaldehyde and borax was used to preserve food . They used Copper Sulphate to make pickles greener and Red Lead to color candy. Pure poison.

In 1856 Sir William Henry Perkins created the color Mauve from coal tar. (which yellow dye #5 is made from ). By 1900 there were 80 dyes made from coal tar.

While there are no actual statistics, a great many people died from these colors. Around that time, the Chief Chemist of the Dept. of Agriculture, Dr. Henry Washington Wiley was brave enough to publicly declare, "The American people are being steadfastly poisoned by the dangerous chemicals that are being added to food with reckless abandon".[20]

In 1906 Theodore Roosevelt created the Food and Drug Act, which led to the immediate ban of 73 of the 80 coal tar dyes. Many of these proven to be carcinogenic are still being used today. Benzyl Violet #1, used for 22 years in beverages, candy, ice cream, baked goods and cosmetics was finally banned in 1973. Others have come and gone but many of the existing ones (Yellow 5, Yellow 6, Red 3, Red 40, Blue 1, Blue 2, Green 3 ) made from coal tar or petroleum are just as toxic and found to have a direct correlation to behavior problems, learning problems and health problems, including cancer.

The UK and Europe have already banned some Artificial Colors or at least put a Warning Label on the ones still allowed because they have proven that the food dyes are destroying the Behavior and Learning of their children.

Our FDA ( Food and Drug Administration) had a 2 day hearing March 30-31, 2011 to discuss putting Warning Labels on foods containing toxic food dyes. They dragged their feet and decided that more studies were needed.

It is a fact that Artificial Food Colors contain mercury, lead, arsenic and benzidine. The FDA sets a minimum allowed amount of these toxic substances because they know it's impossible to remove the toxins, but random samples tested of Food Dyes have revealed levels up to 100 times higher than the allowed 1ppb. [18]

It's interesting to note that a McDonald's strawberry sundae in Britain is colored with strawberries but in the USA it's Red 40. Fanta soda is colored orange in Britain with pumpkin and carrot extract but the same soda in the USA uses Red 40 and Yellow 6 . Also in Britain, natural colors are used in Starbursts and Skittles but artificial colors are used for the children in America, and we wonder why there's an epidemic of Autistic Spectrum Disorders. [19]

# 21     BAKING SODA and ALKALIZING

I mentioned it before in chapter 6 about brushing your teeth with Baking Soda (sodium bicarbonate) but at that time I didn't realize its other amazing powers. Besides deodorizing, cleaning, and alkalizing pools you can actually reverse a food intolerance reaction by drinking a ½ tsp. baking soda in a half glass of water.  (you can also take 1 tablet of Alka-Aid or 1 Alka Seltzer Gold Antacid ) [17]

If you know that you accidently ate something you shouldn't have, you can even prevent the reaction by alkalizing with one of the above.  ( reactions can be physical or behavioral ). This does not mean that you should purposely eat and drink things you react to and then take baking soda and water everyday.

When a person overdoses on aspirin (acetyl salicylic acid ) they are rushed to the hospital,  have their stomach pumped,  and are put on an IV of Sodium Bicarbonate to reverse the effects of a toxic amount of Salicylates. Thus proving the antidotal effects of baking soda on salicylates.

Having a swig of baking soda in water at night before you go to bed is a good antacid for Acid Reflux. It is healing to the esophagus at night when you lie down, but doesn't reduce the acid during the day when you need acid to digest your food. Other medications decrease your acid 24/7 and can cause many other problems.

I have actually gotten rid of food induced headaches by taking a swig of baking soda in water as soon as it comes on. The first time I was happily surprised since I wasn't sure it would really work. It's one thing to read about something and another to actually experience it for yourself. So don't believe me, try it !!!!!!

Besides using baking soda, Lemons and Limes squeezed in water are a great way to alkalize our bodies. It is so important to our health to keep our bodies alkalized. Bacteria, Viruses Fungi and Cancer thrive in an acidic environment. They can't grow in an alkalized body.

The most acidic foods are: Sugar, Artificial Sweeteners, Alcohol, Soda, Meat, and Cheese. To alkalize drink lemon/limes in water and eat whatever fruits or vegetables agree with you.

Years ago I read a book called "Alkalize or Die". It was pretty scary, need I say

more.

# 22 CELIAC, GLUTEN INTOLERANCE and HISTAMINE

I am not an expert in Celiac Disease but I have a good understanding of Gluten Intolerance and NCGS ( non celiac gluten sensitivity ). Gluten is in wheat, barley and rye.

Celiac Disease causes a person to be so intolerant to gluten that even trace amounts can cause severe damage to the villi in their intestines. Once damaged they stop producing certain enzymes necessary to properly digest food. Something called Leaky Gut can develop allowing gluten and other undigested food to enter the bloodstream. The body then sees this as an attack by a foreign substance and we can have an allergic reaction.

Allergic reactions go beyond diarrhea and constipation. They can be anything from headaches , hives, eczema, asthma, arthritis to ADHD, Asperger's and other neurological symptoms.

During an allergic reaction the body produces Histamine to fight off an infection or what it believes to be an intruder. Many of us who are

Food/Chemical Sensitive are not good at ridding the body of histamine so it builds up and presents itself simply as sneezing, watery eyes, a cough or runny nose or more serious symptoms such as hives, headaches or asthma. [20] If histamine goes to the brain it clogs up the countless chemical and electrical processes and interferes with normal brain activity. This can affect learning and behavior.

All of the above symptoms caused by histamine are not just a reaction to Celiac but can also be triggered by Salicylate Intolerance, and artificial colors and additives.

Several years ago, after getting rid of all my major symptoms from Salicylate Intolerance I was still experiencing some stomachaches, gas and bloating. I was tested for Celiac, but the results were negative. That's when my doctor told me that people who don't have Celiac could very well have NCGS ( non celiac gluten sensitivity). He said that all humans are sensitive to wheat. Well, that day I cut out bread, pasta and all wheat. I also found that I'm sensitive to barley but not rye.

The bloating subsided and I lost a few pounds. I feel much better avoiding wheat even though I do cheat occasionally. Here's the difference, a person with Celiac can't cheat without instant intestinal damage. If I cheat I get instant gas and bloating.

The last piece to the puzzle for me was also avoiding milk, cheese and ice cream (something I am addicted to and ate every night for 20 years ). I found that it was giving me a very dry mouth in addition to the gas. I'm sure the sugar and corn syrup in the ice cream was part of my problem too. I knew that I was Lactose Intolerant but why was Lactaid Milk and Lactaid Cottage Cheese still giving me gas ? It's possible that I am also sensitive to Casein, the protein in milk.

Avoiding dairy has also helped improve my hemorrhoid problem.

Bottom line, they say that Gluten Intolerance is the Mother of all Food Intolerances. And the Gut (large intestine) is our largest Immune System. If we heal the Gut by avoiding gluten, the other Intolerances could improve or at least become less severe.

# 23    MISCELLANEOUS TOPICS

WATER AND SALT FOR ASTHMA

A small glass of water followed by a pinch (1/16 tsp.) of salt on the tongue afterwards is an old fashion remedy for Asthma. Sodium is a NATURAL MUCOUS BREAKER. The pinch of salt on tongue AFTER drinking the water fools the brain into thinking that the body released salt to make the mucous disposable. The bronchioles relax within 5 minutes making it easier to breath.[21]

I use this whenever I seem to have thick phlegm in my throat making me cough or short of breath. It works every time and it's a lot less expensive than Mucinex.

## ANTIBIOTICS AND PROBIOTICS

When my sons were babies I never gave them an Antibiotic without also giving them a Probiotic. I would open up a capsule of Acidophilus/Lactobacillus and sprinkle it on their tongue. Back then I knew that antibiotics could cause yeast infections and diarrhea and I read that taking a Probiotic would prevent it. I was on to something much bigger. I didn't realize that I was preventing my babies from getting yeast overgrowth in their whole bodies, especially the intestines.

When you take an Antibiotic you are killing all the bacteria in your body including the good bacteria. We need the good bacteria in our intestines to prevent the yeast from growing out of control. If we don't replace the good bacteria by taking Acidophilus, (probiotic) the yeast takes over causing diarrhea, rashes, thrush and possibly Leaky Gut Syndrome. Yeast has tentacles that can work their way through the walls of the intestines. Undigested food escapes through the holes causing all kinds of allergic reactions.

Something even worse can occur , Clostridium Difficile. (C Diff) When we take

an antibiotic without taking a probiotic it kills off all the bacteria except the

VERY WORST, C Diff.  Without good bacteria in the intestines to fight it off,

the  C Diff  takes over, causing fever, severe diarrhea, and terrible body

cramps in the chest and back. At that point it's too late for a simple probiotic

capsule to cure you. In the Hospital they have to treat you with very strong

antibiotics to kill the C Diff and heavy doses of Probiotics to replenish the

good bacteria.

So lesson to be learned: Always take a Probiotic 2 or 3 times a day when on

an Antibiotic and continue taking the next 2 weeks after because an

antibiotic stays in your system at least a week after you are done taking it.

Probiotics can be bought in the Pharmacy near the vitamins.

I actually take a Acidophilus every day or 2 to constantly replenish the good

bacteria to stay healthy. You could eat yogurt but you would have to eat a lot

to get the same amount of acidophilus you get in 1 capsule.

EPSOM SALTS

While I don't soak my feet in Epsom Salt and water very often, some people swear by it. Epsom Salt is Magnesium Sulfate. Many people with Food Intolerances are low in Sulfates which are necessary to properly metabolize Salicylates.

It is important to start out with a small spoonful of Epsom Salt in a small footbath of water to soak your feet. (soaking your feet is just as beneficial as taking a bath in it) I made the mistake of soaking in a cupful of Epsom salts in my bath. When I got out I was very dizzy and nauseous.

In laymen's terms, if we are low in sulfates then our receptors are wide open trying to absorb the low level of sulfates we have. When we soak in Epsom Salts we suddenly have a large supply of sulfates and we could take too much in. Many people on the Salicylatesensitivity.com forum have said that soaking their feet in Epsom salt helps to counteract their symptoms and helps them sleep better.

## DRY MOUTH

While most of my other symptoms disappeared once avoiding Salicylates, I am still plagued with Dry Mouth. I don't take any medication and they ruled out Sjogrens. (which can cause dry mouth and eyes)

In the past I always got a dry mouth after I drank tea or rode in a car. I don't drink tea anymore (high in sals) but driving in a car still makes my mouth dry. There is Benzene and other odorless fumes in a car that can cause reactions in people who are Multiple Chemical Sensitive (MCS). It could be the carpet, the leather, adhesives, mold or other petroleum fumes. Every time I drove in my husbands BMW I got an instant headache. A car dealer said the same thing happened to his wife in his BMW.

Last summer, though, I developed am EXTREMELY DRY MOUTH that lasted for 5 months. By extreme I mean no saliva all day. Dry teeth, dry gums, dry tongue, dry lips, unbearable. One-by-one I eliminated these things trying to find the cause:1) Canola Oil and Rice Vinegar on salad, 2) brushing teeth with hydrogen peroxide, 3) brushing teeth with baking soda, 4) baby oil on skin, 5) very cold, dry air conditioning . Nothing helped.

I went to several doctors to make sure there wasn't a problem with my Saliva Glands or Adrenal Glands. Everything was normal.

It was discovered that my Blood Sugar Level was a little high. By high I mean higher than normal but pre-pre-diabetic (5.9). And I did notice that my dry mouth got worse when I ate a lot of sugar. I also knew that I was Lactose Intolerant but chose to ignore that because it only gave me a little gas, bloating and stomach ache. I have eaten ice cream every night for the past 20 years. Even though I used Lactaid Milk on my cereal in the morning it still didn't agree with me. Perhaps I am also sensitive to CASEIN, the protein in milk.

At this point I had already given up Salicylates and Gluten. So now I decided to give up Dairy. Once I gave up my ice cream at night and bowl of cereal in the morning my chronic dry mouth started to improve. It is interesting to note that we don't have fluoride in our water at home but we do have it at our Shore house. My dry mouth gets worse down the shore so the FLUORIDE could be part of the problem. I still live with some dryness, but it's on and off, not constant. And it is definitely triggered when I drive in a car or eat sugar.

## BURNING LIPS AND TONGUE

This is a new symptom and separate from dry mouth. This also started last summer and is definitely triggered by food.

In addition to the burning/tingling I sometimes get tiny red spots on the top border of my top lip and a tiny bit of swelling. I will also get small flat pink bumps in the front and on top of my tongue. Perhaps these are hives but they have never progressed to anything dangerous like anaphylaxis, thank God.

Last summer I started eating a lot of cabbage because it is low in Sals and I love it. I have a tendency to overdue things. I had raw green cabbage and red cabbage everyday in a salad with papaya, pecans, and feta cheese with canola oil and rice vinegar. Delicious and healthy but too much of a good thing is bad. Cabbage is also a natural blood thinner so you should limit your intake if you are on a blood thinner. After several months of Burning Tongue Syndrome I read that the Cruciferous vegetables (cabbage, broccoli, cauliflower and brussel sprouts) contain a chemical called ISOTHIOCYANATE which can affect the mucous membranes.

When I stopped eating cabbage for awhile the Burning Tongue and Lips greatly improved. I still experience a slight tingling tongue occasionally from a few other foods but not as constant or as bad as last summer. Now I eat cabbage 3 times a week.

DRY CRUSTY SCABBY BLOODY NOSE

Last Summer was full of surprises. I suddenly had a very dry itchy nose full of scabs and occasional bleeding. I tried opening windows instead of drying out the air with air conditioning but that didn't help. I went to the ENT (Ear,Nose,Throat) Doctor and he actually cauterized one side of my nose, but that didn't help either. He gave me a cortisone nasal spray, which had a warning not to use if you had any open sores in your nose.  Duh? My nose

was filled with them so I didn't use it.

Guess what ?  Since the nose is also a mucous membrane, as soon as I gave up

cabbage everyday (with Isothiocyanate) my nose cleared up 100 %.  I can

now tolerate cabbage once or twice a week .

MULTIPLE CHEMICAL SENSITIVITY (MCS )

People who are Salicylate Sensitive (SS) are usually MCS. My first real

Asthma attack was triggered after spraying bug spray in my son's room for

spiders.  Another one happened after spraying Lysol on my mattress.

I had to get rid of a brand new Tempurpedic mattress because it was emitting

petroleum gasses. As soon as they set it up I became dizzy and was having

trouble breathing.  They had to remove it the same day they delivered it.

Riding in a car makes my mouth dry and sometimes gives me a headache. All

the dyes, fumes and cleaning products in a mall or food store makes my eyes

irritated and bloodshot and I get a foggy headed feeling.  And why do they always have to spray windex on the table next to me in the restaurant when I am eating ? Ugh !

MCS people are affected by other peoples' perfume, room deodorizers and scents in lotions and hand soap. We have to use fragrance-free and dye-free shampoos, fabric softening sheets, and clothes detergents.

Children are affected by spray deodorant, bus fumes, parents' cigarette smoke, dry erase markers, fluoride in water and gasses emitted from new furniture, carpeting, newly painted walls and many other chemicals. It can affect their health, learning and behavior.

# 24 LIST OF SYMPTOMS of SALICYLATE INTOLERANCE

The list on the next page is a compilation of symptoms formed after studying 10 different lists off the Internet. It's possible to only have 2 or 3 of the symptoms but some people have many more[3, 4, 11]. There is one list that cites 133 ailments attributable to Salicylate Intolerance. I think that might be pushing it so I've only listed the most common symptoms. Notice how many of these are similar to Fibromyalgia symptoms. Hmm, I bet most people diagnosed with Fibromyalgia are actually Salicylate Intolerant. Much of the information on Salicylate Intolerance originated from the Feingold Association. (See http://www.feingold.org) Remember, these symptoms occur because you are walking around in a constant state of inflammation somewhere in your body (brain, joints, bronchioles etc.) as a result of a toxic overload of Salicylates, Artificial Colors, Preservatives and other Chemicals in your body.

# SYMPTOMS OF SALICYLATE INTOLERANCE

Migraines

Red eyes

Burning eyes

Dry eyes

Watery eyes

Pain and pressure in eye

Eye muscle disorders

Eye muscle pain

Vision problems

Crossed eyes

Drifting eye

Hives

Mental sluggishness

Upset stomach

Bloody noses

Nasal polyps

Sinusitis

Nasal congestion

Diarrhea

Hemorrhoids

Hot flash/chills

Flushing

Swelling of Saliva Glands

Swelling of lips, eyes & face

Burning lips

Mouth sores

Canker sores

Persistent cough

Pain in joints

Arthritis

Chronic fatigue

Vertigo

Foggy headed

Difficulty focusing

ADHD

Easily distracted

Fidgetiness

Nervousness

Anaphylaxis

Anxiety

Constipation

Restless Leg Syndrome

Itchy skin and scalp

Rashes,  Hives

Changes in skin color

Bloated stomach

Thirst

Urge to urinate often

Depression, irritability

Temper flare-ups

Inability to concentrate

Ringing in ear

Pain in ear

Pinching / swelling in ear

Pressure across forehead

Very dry mouth

Pinchy sore throat

Itchy throat and tongue

Meniere's Disease

Eczema

| | | |
|---|---|---|
| Autism 23 | Seizures | PDD |
| Fibromyalgia | Dyslexia | Acid Reflux |
| Hypoglycemia | Chronic Back Pain | IBS |
| Bi-Polar Disorder | Heart Palpitations | Tourette's |
| Bedwetting | Tinnitus | Throat clearing |
| Glue ear(thick wax) | Panic Attacks | Aggression (ODD) |
| Ear Infections | Dark Circles under eyes | OCD |
| Sleep Problems | Speech Problems | Thick Phlegm in throat |
| Fever/Chills | Swollen Feet/ankles/hands | Heavy Periods |

# 25 FOOD GUIDE
## Fruits

| NEGLIGIBLE | LOW | MODERATE | HIGH | VERY HIGH |
|---|---|---|---|---|
| Banana | Apple-golden Delicious | Apple-red Delicious | Apple-Tart | All dried fruits |
| Pear (peeled) | Nashi Pears | Canned Fig | Granny Smith | Apricot |
| Canned Pear ( in light syrup) | Papaya | Fresh Figs | Canned cherries | Avocado |
| Lime | | Custard Apple | Cantaloupe | All Berries |
| | | Lemon | Dried Figs | Blackberries |
| | | Loquat | Grapefruit | Blackcurrant |
| | | Mango | Kiwi | Blueberry |
| | | Passion fruit | Lychee | Boysenberry |
| | | Paw Paw | Mandarins | Cherries |
| | | Pear (with peel) | Melons | Cranberry |
| | | Persimmon | Mulberry | Currant |
| | | Pomegranate | Nectarine | Date |
| | | Tamarillo | Peach | Grape |
| | | | Rhubarb | Guava |
| | | | Sugar Banana | Loganberry |

| NEGLIGIBLE | LOW | MODERATE | HIGH | VERY HIGH |
|---|---|---|---|---|
| | | | Watermelon | Orange |
| | | | | Pineapple |
| | | | | Plum |
| | | | | Prune |
| | | | | Raisin |
| | | | | Raspberry |
| | | | | Redcurrant |
| | | | | Rock Melon |
| | | | | Strawberry |
| | | | | Sultana |
| | | | | Tangelo |
| | | | | Tangerine |
| | | | | Youngberry |
| | | | | |

# Vegetables

| NEGLIGIBLE | LOW | MODERATE | HIGH | VERY HIGH |
|---|---|---|---|---|
| Bamboo shoots | Bean sprouts | Asparagus (fresh or can) | Alfalfa sprouts | Green olives |
| | Borlotti Beans | | Artichoke | Capsicum |
| Beans (dried, fresh or canned) | Brussel sprouts | Aubergine (peeled) | Aubergine (with peel) | Champignon |
| Cabbage (green or white) | Cabbage (red) | Beets (fresh or canned) | Broad Bean | Chicory |
| | Chickpeas | | | |
| Celery | Chives | | Broccoli | Chili Peppers |
| Green split peas | Choko | Black olives | Carrots | Endive |
| Lentils (red or brown) | String beans | Cauliflower | Corn (fresh or canned) | Gherkin pickles |
| | Green onions | Fresh tomato | Cucumber | All peppers |
| Lettuce (iceberg) | Green peas (fresh or canned) | Frozen spinach | Eggplant | Hot peppers |
| Peas (dried) | Leek | Lettuce (other than iceberg) | Fresh Spinach | Jalapenos peppers |
| Potato (old, white, & peeled) | Potato (not peeled) | Turnips | Okra | Radish |
| Swede | Shallots | Mushrooms | Pickled beets | Tomato |
| | Yellow split peas | Onion | Red pepper | Anything tomato |

| NEGLIGIBLE | LOW | MODERATE | HIGH | VERY HIGH |
|---|---|---|---|---|
| | | Parsnips | Squash | Water chestnuts |
| | | Romaine | Sweet potato | |
| | | Potato<br>(new & red Pontiac) | Watercress | |
| | | | Zucchini | Pimientos |
| | | Pumpkin | | |
| | | Snow peas | | |
| | | Sweet corn | | |

# Nuts and Seeds

| Negligible | Low | Moderate | High | Very high |
|---|---|---|---|---|
| Poppy seed | Cashews | Desiccated coconut | Brazil nuts | Almond |
| | Hazelnuts | Peanut butter | Macadamia | Peanut with skin on |
| | Pecans | Pumpkin seeds | Pine nuts | Water chestnuts |
| | Sunflower seeds | Walnuts | Pistachio | |
| | | | Sesame seeds | |
| | | | Tahini | |

# Sweets

| Negligible | Low | Moderate | High | Very high |
|---|---|---|---|---|
| Carob | Caramel | Molasses | | Chewing Gum |
| Maple Syrup | Golden Syrup | Raw Sugar | | Fruit Flavors |
| White Sugar | Malt Extract | | | Honey |
| | | | | Honey Flavors |
| | | | | Jam (except pear) |
| | | | | Licorice |
| | | | | All mint flavored sweets |
| | | | | Peppermints |

# Seasonings, Condiments, Sauces, and Toppings

| Negligible | Low | Moderate | High | Very High |
|---|---|---|---|---|
| Malt Vinegar | Homemade Apple Butter | Fresh Coriander | All Spice | Aniseed |
| Maple Syrup | Chives | Chinese Parsley | Bay Leaf | Basil |
| Rice Vinegar | Fennel –dried | Horseradish | Caraway | Black Pepper |
| Salt | Garlic | Mayonnaise | Cardamom | Cayenne |
| | Parsley | | Cloves | Cinnamon |
| | Saffron | | Coriander | Celery Powder |
| | Shallots | | Mixed Herbs | Chili Flakes |
| | Soy Sauce (not low sodium) | | Pimiento | Chili Powder |
| | Sake Rice Wine | | | Apple Cider Vinegar |
| | Mirin Sweet Rice Wine | | | Commercial Gravy and Sauces |
| | | | | Cumin |
| | | | | Curry |
| | | | | Dill |
| | | | | Dried Mustard |

| NEGLIGIBLE | LOW | MODERATE | HIGH | VERY HIGH |
|---|---|---|---|---|
| | | | | Fenugreek |
| | | | | Ginger |
| | | | | Honey |
| | | | | All commercial jam and jelly |
| | | | | Ketchup |
| | | | | Jalapeno & Buffalo |
| | | | | Mace |
| | | | | Marmite |
| | | | | Mint |
| | | | | Mustard |
| | | | | Nutmeg |
| | | | | Oregano |
| | | | | Paprika |
| | | | | Peppermint |
| | | | | Rosemary |
| | | | | Sage |
| | | | | Spearmint |
| | | | | Tabasco Hot Sauce |

| NEGLIGIBLE | LOW | MODERATE | HIGH | VERY HIGH |
|---|---|---|---|---|
| | | | | Tarragon |
| | | | | Tomato Paste |
| | | | | Tomato Powder |
| | | | | Thyme |
| | | | | Turmeric |
| | | | | Vegemite and other yeast extracts |
| | | | | Wasabi |
| | | | | White Pepper |
| | | | | White Vinegar |
| | | | | Wintergreen (Can be toxic to someone who is Salicylate Intolerant)15 |
| | | | | Worcestershire Sauce |
| | | | | Wine Vinegar |

# Fats and Oils

| Negligible | Low | Moderate | High | Very High |
|---|---|---|---|---|
| Butter | Ghee | Almond Oil | Copha | Coconut Oil |
| Canola Oil | | Corn Oil | Sesame Oil | OLIVE OIL |
| Margerine | | Peanut Oil | Walnut Oil | |
| Safflower Oil | | | | |
| Soy Oil | | | | |
| Sunflower oil | | | | |

# Grains

| Negligible | Low | Moderate | High | Very High |
|---|---|---|---|---|
| Barley | | | | Cereal w/ Almonds, Fruit, Honey, or Coconut |
| Buckwheat | | | | Corn Cereal |
| Millet | | | | Flavored Cereal |
| Oats | | | | Maize |
| Rice | | | | Polenta |
| Rice Cereal | | | | Cornmeal |
| Rye | | | | |
| Wheat | | | | |

# Meat

| Negligible | Low | Moderate | High | Very High |
|---|---|---|---|---|
| Beef | Liver | | Fish canned with unacceptable oil | Processed Luncheon Meat with spices |
| Chicken | Prawns | | Gravy from bouillon cubes or mixes | Seasoned Meats (e.g. salami, sausages) |

| NEGLIGIBLE | LOW | MODERATE | HIGH | VERY HIGH |
|---|---|---|---|---|
| Eggs | Shellfish | | Bacon | Anchovies |
| Fish | Shrimp | | Chicken Liver | Fish Roe |
| Lamb | | | Ham | Hot Dogs |
| Organ Meat | | | Oysters | Smoked Meat |
| Rabbit | | | Pork | Canned Tuna in Oil |
| Sausage casing | | | Salmon | |
| Scallops | | | Sardines | |
| Tripe | | | Fresh Tuna | |
| Veal | | | | |

# Dairy and Soy Products

| Negligible | Low | Moderate | High | Very High |
|---|---|---|---|---|
| Butter | | Blue Vein Cheese | | |
| Cream | | Blue Cheese | | |
| Cheese ( not blue vein ) | | Gorgonzola | | |
| Milk | | | | |
| Yogurt | | | | |
| Ice Cream | | | | |
| Rice Milk | | | | |
| Goat Milk | | | | |
| Soy Milk | | | | |
| Tofu | | | | |

# Baking Supplies

| Negligible | Low | Moderate | High | Very High |
|---|---|---|---|---|
| Arrowroot | | Sesame Seeds | Corn Syrup | Honey |
| Corn Starch | | | | Vanilla |
| Cocoa | | | | |
| Golden Syrup | | | | |
| Malt | | | | |
| Malt Extract | | | | |
| Poppy Seeds | | | | |
| Rice Flour | | | | |
| Rye Flour | | | | |
| Sago | | | | |
| Soy Flour | | | | |
| Sugar | | | | |
| Sugar (Brown, castor, granulated ) | | | | |
| Powdered sugar and icing | | | | |
| Tapioca | | | | |
| Wheat Flour | | | | |

# Commercial Snacks

| Negligible | Low | Moderate | High | Very High |
|---|---|---|---|---|
| | Plain Potato chips | Apple Chips (homemade from acceptable types) | Popcorn | Chewing Gum (all flavors) |
| | | | | Fruit flavored Candy, Gelato,Ices,Popsicles, Sherbet, Sorbet,and Sweets |
| | | | | Licorice/Liquorices |
| | | | | All Flavors |
| | | | | Mints, Peppermint, Spearmint and Wintergreen (toxic) |
| | | | | Flavored Gum and Candy |
| | | | | Pickles (anything pickled) |
| | | | | |

# Beverages

Beverages to avoid: All Tea, peppermint tea, green tea, spearmint tea, brewed coffee, all fruit juice, soda, carbonated drinks, V-8 juice, Beer, Wine, Sherry, Brandy, and Rum.

Acceptable Beverages: WATER, ice water, hot water, water with lemon, water with lime, Milk, Postum, Instant decaf coffee, vodka, gin, scotch whiskey and sake.
(I still get a headache from Instant decaf coffee)

# 26 FOOD JOURNAL AND STUPID MISTAKES

These are all mistakes I made eating foods that were high in Salicylates. Some I didn't realize till after I got sick and some challenges I made fully aware but hoping that I could tolerate them.

Sept.2007 – We went out for dinner with friends. I had a Vodka and Tonic (Tonic is quinine which I can't tolerate. It's in coffee and cranberry juice also.) For dinner I ate a Pasta with mushrooms, artichoke hearts, shrimp, wine and olive oil. I thought I was doing good by not having tomato sauce.  At the end of the meal I had a decaf coffee.

I had a Migraine as we were leaving.  It lasted all night.  At 5:30 am I woke up with severe Vertigo. The room was spinning.  It was worse if I tried to lie back down. I threw up for 2 hours then sat up in a chair for an hour trying to sleep. At 9:00 a.m. I tried to eat breakfast and as the day went on I started feeling better.

March 2008 – The restaurant didn't have ranch dressing for my salad so I put a little Olive oil on it but no vinegar. I said to my husband, "Watch, I bet I wake up with bloodshot eyes tomorrow "and sure enough I did. I looked like Dracula. My husband couldn't believe it.

April 2008 – I used to love coffee. But now I have confirmed that every time I have a cup of decaf coffee I get a headache in my eyes. I never made the connection before. They say that decaf instant coffee has less Salicylates. Chocolate also gives me a headache as well as MSG.

April 23, 2008 – I went to my friend's house after work. Everybody had a Margarita. I decided to try a Virgin Margarita with no alcohol. I got the worst migraine that lasted all night. The next day I looked at the ingredients. Margarita Mix has Yellow dye #5 and High Fructose Corn Syrup.

July 2008 – I painted my bedroom. That night I had sticky bloodshot eyes from the fumes.

July 11, 2008 – I was fine all day. At night I had ice cream with a lot of Hot Fudge. I got a bad headache in my eyes.

July 20, 2008 – I had mustard on my sandwich, honey wheat bread, and some ice cream later. Something I ate gave me sticky bloodshot eyes.

Aug.6, 2008 – Something gave me terrible Vertigo. (Dizziness) I ate some avocado on my sandwich. I ate stuffed Grape leaves cooked with mint and I had a piece of banana bread made with *Splenda*. It all adds up.

Aug.20, 2008 -- My eyes have been really clear for awhile now. Today I tried a peeled apple and had a chicken burrito with spicy cheese sauce on it. I woke up with very bloodshot eyes.

Aug.27, 2008 - We went to a friend's house for a party. They had Tortellini salad with olive oil and vinegar, Sausage and peppers with tomato sauce; mozzarella and tomato salad drizzled with balsamic vinegar, eggplant parmigiana, (parmesan cheese) shrimp and tomato salad with olive oil and vinegar, and cheeseburgers. I thought I would be safe with a cheeseburger till I took the first bite. It tasted too good, so I asked what was in the meat. They had mixed ketchup in the meat before cooking it. I HAD A ROLL AND BUTTER FOR DINNER AT THE PARTY.

Sept.1, 2008 - Tonight I am foggy headed, I have a headache, my neck hurts more than usual and my lips burn. Today at a funeral dinner I chose the shrimp over linguini since everything else had tomato sauce on it. It must have been made with olive oil. I also had a *Cinnabon* which is obviously made with cinnamon.  AT ITALIAN RESTAURANTS I

ORDER GARLIC SAUTEED IN BUTTER OVER PASTA AND I PUT PARMIGIANO

CHEESE ON IT.  It's safe and delicious.

Sept 27, 2008 – I baked brussel sprouts with red cabbage and onions. I just had to tempt

fate with a few peeled and cut up apples in it. Of course I got a sore throat, swollen

glands, foggy headed and achy.  When will I learn?  I'm almost done writing this book

and I'm still testing my tolerance for foods.

Oct.21, 2008 - I was fine all day. For dinner I had several pieces of precooked and

vacuum packed Roast Beef. I am supposed to have very fresh meat. Supposedly as meat

ages something called AMINES multiplies and can make you sick if you are sensitive to

it.   I woke up with sticky bloodshot eyes, very achy neck and joints and inflamed

hemorrhoids.

Oct.30, 2008 - This is the last journal entry I am going to write because this is the mother

of all mistakes I've made.  Last night I had dinner at Applebee's. I ordered Lime Fiesta

Chicken without the tomatoes on top and I told the waiter, no paprika on anything.  It

came with rice on the side.   Earlier in the day I also had another piece of the precooked

roast beef (not too smart).

I went to school the next day feeling fine.  By 3<sup>rd</sup> period I was achy all over and had chills.  By 4<sup>th</sup> period I was nauseas and felt like I was going to faint.  I got tingly all over and my mouth went totally dry.  One of the students ran to get the other Art Teacher.  She called for the nurse.  I couldn't walk because I was so dizzy and nauseas.  They took me to the nurse's office in a wheel chair and since I couldn't drive home, my son picked me up.  The nurse said she sent 3 kids home with the same virus that day. So I thought maybe it was a virus.  Then the muscles in my eyes started to hurt and I knew exactly what I had.  I went home, got in bed and slept it off.  I called Applebee's that night and found out that the Mexican Rice had dried tomato powder, chili powder and extract of paprika.  BINGO!!!  Poison Pilaf.

Lastly, in my continuing research, I just read that soaking your feet in Epsom Salts or taking a warm (not hot) bath in it can help reduce the salicylate toxins in your body. It is suggested that you rinse off in a cool shower after the bath.

It's not easy.  I still make mistakes. Try to avoid all the foods in the High and Extremely High column and you will start to feel better. At least I have many more good days than bad now. And when I have a bad day at least now I can figure out why.

# 27 SUGGESTED MEALS and SOME RECIPES

## BREAKFAST

**High Fiber Cereal with Lactaid Milk – (Cheerios, Grape Nuts, Smart Start, Special K, Rice Chex)**

**Oatmeal**

**Banana with Sunflower Butter or Chocolate Hazelnut Spread. (Not Nutella it has Vanillin in it)  I found an A&P brand that uses real vanilla in it.**

**Eggs (any style) – Poached, over easy, or scrambled with cheese. NO KETCHUP**

**Or my favorite, Poached Eggs over Rice or over Quinoa.**

**Bacon or Taylor Ham in very small doses (because of the Sodium Nitrate)**

**Pancakes with butter and real Maple Syrup or powdered sugar. (Fake maple syrup is corn syrup )**

**Bagel with butter, or Lox or cream cheese, or egg and cheese.**

# LUNCH

## The only spices I use are salt, garlic, lemon and parsley

IF SENSITIVE TO AMINES EAT ONLY FRESH MEAT and FISH and AVOID COLD CUTS, BACON and aged cheeses.

Sandwich – Boars Head ham or roast beef. (sometimes turkey has paprika on outside for color)

Swiss cheese, mozzarella, white American (not yellow –yellow dye #5)

On Arnold Country Wheat bread. (some multi grain breads have raisin juice, high fructose corn syrup, sesame seeds or almonds) with lettuce and mayonnaise.

Grilled Cheese

Cheeseburger with lettuce and mayonnaise (mayo has some vinegar in it but I am able to tolerate a little since I can't have mustard or ketchup )

Fish sandwich with lettuce and mayonnaise. (No Cocktail sauce,  No Tartar sauce , it has chopped pickles in it )

White Pasta Fagiola – (no olive oil, no tomato sauce) sauté beans in butter, add chicken broth, pasta, parmesan cheese and parsley.

New England clam chowder (white, nothing pink and avoid MSG)

Split Pea Soup

Can of peas,(peas are high on some lists) Can of string beans (or fresh or frozen )

Celery with Sunflower Butter.

Tuna fish salad with celery (no onions )

Egg salad (no onions )

 Chicken salad (no onions)

Tuna mixed with egg salad or Chicken salad mixed with egg salad.

 Sunflower Seed Butter, Cashew butter, pecan butter or walnut butter and banana sandwich on Rice cake

White pizza(make sure they don't put olive oil in the dough).

Calzone with cheese (no tomato sauce )

Salad – just lettuce, cabbage, celery, pecans or walnuts, papaya, and cheese with canola oil and rice vinegar or a little ranch dressing.

Beans over brown rice or Quinoa.

Chinese food – (careful of too much ginger, red pepper, and corn starch)

I seem to be ok with: Chicken and string beans over rice

Shrimp and string beans

Shrimp in lobster sauce

Chicken LoMein

SUSHI – any fish with asparagus (no cucumbers or avocados) use regular soy sauce,

(no Low Sodium soy sauce, it contains vinegar)

# DINNER

**Steak** – salt and garlic powder (no spicy seasoning)

**Chicken** – grilled, breaded and fried, or baked with Canola oil and breadcrumbs

**Chicken Francaise** – dipped in flour, eggs, breadcrumbs, sauté in butter and lemon juice.

**(no wine or olive oil )**

**Shrimp Scampi** – Garlic, butter, lemon, salt and parsley (No olive oil or wine)
**No lemon pepper with yellow dye #5 or Turmeric.**

**PASTA** - sauté garlic in butter, mix in with pasta and parmesan cheese.

**Sautéed cabbage in butter, garlic salt, parsley, over egg noodles. (mix in sour cream)**

**Caesar Salad** – (no Caesar dressing) Ranch dressing on the side.

**Garlic bread with mozzarella and Parmesan cheese (no oregano)**

**Steamed Lobster dipped in butter with lemon (no paprika)**

**Clams** – Raw, steamed, or grilled with melted butter (no cocktail sauce)

**Roasted Brussel sprouts or Cabbage wedges. ( or some cauliflower, it's moderate)**

# DESSERTS

**DON'T OVERDUE IT. THERE ARE HIDDEN ARTIFICIAL FLAVORS, COLORS, PRESERVATIVES, AND HIGH FRUCTOSE CORN SYRUP.**

**Breyers natural vanilla or chocolate ice cream   (no almonds, no fruit flavors)**

**Whip cream**

**Flan**

**Pudding –Cook and Serve ( Instant has too many artificial colors, flavors and preservatives )**

**Cake**

**Cookies**

**Cheesecake**

# BEVERAGES

**WATER- Ice water with lemon or lime, cup of Hot water.**

**Scotch and water,    Vodka over ice with lime, Sake rice wine**

**Club Soda or Seltzer**

**NO coffee, NO tea , NO soda, NO wine, NO beer, NO fruit juice.**

# SOME RECIPES

## Alfredo Sauce

Garlic salt with parsley

4 tbsp. butter

2 rounded tbsp. flour

2 cups milk

1 cup parmesan cheese

Melt butter, stir in flour, shake in garlic salt, stir in milk.   Bring to boil while stirring.

When it thickens lower heat and stir in Parmesan cheese. Take off heat and cover.

# Apple Dessert

9 yellow delicious apples, peeled and cut in chunks        Put in pot

Cover with water (about 3 cups) Add 3 tbsp. brown sugar or real maple syrup

Bring to boil. Simmer for 18 Min.

Add 4 tbsp. Kraft Minute Tapioca. Stir in for 3 minutes. Turn off heat, let cool

Dessert will  thicken more as it cools.

# Lemon Garlic Shrimp (Scampi)

1 Bag frozen or fresh shrimp (cleaned)          4  Tbsp.Canola oil

Garlic salt with parsley  (spoonful chopped garlic optional)

4 Tbsp. butter                                  1 Tbsp. lemon juice

Saute' fresh or frozen shrimp in Canola oil with chopped garlic.  Shake in garlic salt with parsley. Stir in butter, squeeze in lemon juice.  Serve over brown rice or pasta.


# White Lasagna

1 pkg. lasagna noodles (preboil)                1 ½ cups parmesan cheese

1 container ricotta (2 or 3 lb.)                1 pkg. shredded mozzarella

3 eggs                                          1 tbsp. garlic salt with parsley

4 tbsp. butter                                  2 cups milk

Melt butter and pour in milk and ½ cup of Parmesan cheese. Set aside.

Mix ricotta, eggs, 1 cup Parmesan, pkg. of mozzarella and garlic salt.

Layer noodles, ricotta, noodles, ricotta, noodles and sprinkle with Parmesan.

Pour milk with butter and cheese all over the top.  Cover and BAKE at 350 for 1 hour.

# Turkey Rice Alfredo

1 lb.chopped beef or turkey

1 cup brown rice cooked (makes 4 cups)

¾ cups Parmesan cheese or ½ cup Feta

4 tbsp.butter

1 ¼ cups milk or half & half

Garlic salt with parsley

Pre cook rice, put aside to cool. Brown chop meat in pan, sprinkle on garlic salt to taste.

Add 4 tbsp. butter, melt and stir. Add milk, stir. Add Parmesan, stir. Add cooked rice, stir.

If desired, add can of peas.

# Baked Chicken

Line chicken pieces in baking pan.  Sprinkle with garlic salt and Italian breadcrumbs.  Drizzle with about a cup of Canola oil.  Bake at 350 . White meat 50 minutes.    Dark meat 1 hour.

# Chicken Salad

Large can Chicken or fresh cut up.  2 large hard boiled eggs chopped up. Cut up Celery and Red cabbage. Add Mayonaise, salt, garlic powder.

# Greek Moussaka

Modified with no tomato paste, no wine and no eggplant.  Bake 50 min. at 350

| | |
|---|---|
| 4 Tbsp. butter | 1 lb. chop meat |
| 1 tbsp. dried parsley | 1 tsp. garlic salt |
| 3 eggs (beaten) | 2 cups breadcrumbs |
| 1 cup Parmesan cheese | 5 potatoes (no skin) thinly sliced |

Grease bottom of 9x13 baking dish with Canola oil. Sprinkle thin layer of breadcrumbs in pan. Line bottom with ½ of sliced potatoes.

Melt butter in pan, brown meat in butter, stir in parsley, garlic salt, beaten eggs, breadcrumbs and Parmesan cheese.

Pour meat mixture on top of sliced potatoes in pan and arrange another layer of sliced potatoes on top.

## CRÈME SAUCE

3 Tbsp. butter     ½ cup flour     2 cups milk     3 egg yolks (beaten)     1 cup Parmesan cheese

Melt butter, add flour, stir,  add milk,  stir while heating.

Pour about ½ cup of hot crème sauce into the beaten egg yolks, stir, then pour all of the egg mixture back into the crème sauce.    Add 1 cup Parmesan, stir.

Pour crème sauce on top of potatoes.  Cover.  Bake 50 min. at 350.

# Lemon Garlic Chicken

Put about 20 pieces of frozen chicken tenders in baking dish

Mix : 1cup Canola oil, ¾ cup lemon juice, 1 tbsp.dried parsley, 1 tbsp. chopped garlic, garlic salt to

     taste. Stir and pour over chicken.  Sprinkle and cover top with Italian Breadcrumbs.

Bake at 350 for about 40 minutes.

# Taco Pie

| | |
|---|---|
| 1 can refried beans | 1 lb. chop meat |
| Garlic salt with parsley | 1 bag cheddar cheese |
| 2 soft round flour tortillas (9") | |

Brown meat and season with garlic salt. Spray bottom of pie plate with PAM.  Place one round

tortilla on bottom of pan.  Spread refried beans on tortilla.  Pour browned meat on top of beans.

Pour bag of cheese on top of meat.  Place flour tortilla of top. Bake at 350 for 20 – 25 min. If you are making this for someone else who is not Salicylate Intolerant you can put Taco seasoning in meat and Salsa on top of tortilla before baking.

# Stuffed Cabbage

1 cup rice ( 4 cups when cooked)                    1 lb.chopped beef or turkey

12 leaves off head of cabbage                        garlic salt with parsley

5 tbsp. butter                                        1 tbsp.lemon juice

¼ cup Feta cheese                                    ¾ cup beef or chicken broth

Pre cook rice. Parboil cabbage to loosen leaves and pull off 12. (cut around core to make leaf removal easier)

Mix cooked rice, meat, garlic salt and feta cheese.   Place heaping spoonful of meat rice mixture in each cabbage leaf, roll up, place in baking dish.

Put butter, garlic salt, broth and lemon juice on top.  Cover and bake at 350 for 1 hour.

# Cabbage and Egg Noodles

Cut up half head of cabbage, sauté in 5 Tbsp. butter, sprinkle on garlic salt.

Boil 1 pkg. Egg Noodles, drain, pour cabbage over noodles. Mix in 1 small container Sour Cream if desired.

If you are not too affected by Sodium Nitrate,  you can slice up some Kielbasi and sauté it in with the cabbage.

# Saute'd Tofu

Cut 1 pkg. extra firm Tofu into cubes.  Melt 4 Tbsp. butter in pan.  Pour tofu in pan, sprinkle with garlic salt and sauté.

# Quinoa

1 cup ( or 1 part) Quinoa.   1 ½ cups water ( 1 ½ parts water ).  2 tbsp.canola oil. Add salt and garlic powder to taste.

Cover, bring to boil, simmer for 15 min.  Remove from heat, add a little butter and some parmigiana cheese to taste.

# Banana Cake

1 pkg. White Cake Mix (not yellow with yellow dye #5)

1 ¼ cups water                                    1/3 cup Canola oil

3 eggs                                    5 Tbsp. brown sugar

4 over ripe bananas

Mix cake mix with water, oil and eggs. Mash in bananas with fork. Stir in.  Pour into 9x13 baking dish  sprayed with PAM.  Sprinkle brown sugar on top.  Bake at 350 for 30 min.

# 21 REFERENCES

#1)  Salicylate, Amine and other Food Intolerances -

http://www.users.bigpond.com/mywebhome/sindex.html

#2) Salicylate Sensitivity – All about Salicylates and Salicylate Sensitivity -

http://Salicylatesensitivity.com/food-guide/

#3) Salicylate Intolerance Information : By Cheryl and Doug Atkinson – June 2006

http://magicref.tripod.com/health/salicylate.htm

#4)  Severe Aspirin Induced Asthma – Story 4 – Jan.2003

http://www.fedupwithfoodadditives.info/stories/story4.htm

#5)  Types of Autism; What if it's more complex than Mercury? By Dr.Donna Williams

7/03/07 http://www.americanchronicle.com/articles/viewArticle.asp?articleID=31154

#6) Fluoride, Autism and a Potential Gut Connection – by Dr.Donna Williams 7/22/07

http://www.americanchronicle.com/articles/32731

#7) Guai-Support Group (GG) Information and Support for Fibromyalgia Oct 1997

http://www.psha-inc.com/guai-support/sf/Sal-Free/About_Salicylates.htm

#8) Food Intolerance Network Factsheet SALICYLATES 1/30/07

http://www.fedupwithfoodadditives.info/factsheets/FactSalicylates2.htm

#9) Discovery Health – HEADACHE by Terry Mason  Aug.2000

http://healthdiscovery.com/centers/articles/articles.html?chrome=12&article=LC_17&center=p09

#10) TARTRAZINE modified May 11, 2008

http://en.wikipedia.org/wiki/Tartrazine

#11)  http://www.Salicylatesensitivity.com/about

#12)  http://www.webmd.com/content/article/61/67475

#13)  http://www.foodcanmakeyouill.co.uk/sali/salfood.htm

#14) Salicylates in Food - Edited by Jack Campin Aug.2002

http://www.purr.demon.co.uk/Food/Salicylate.html

#15) Teen Dies from Muscle Cream Overdose (Ben Gay Alert)

http://www.freerepublic.com/focus/f-chat/1847216/posts

#16) Donna William's Blog – Fluoride, gut and metabolic damage and a potential Autism link.

http://blog.donnawilliams.net/2007/07/20/fluoride-gut-and-metabolic-damage-and-a-potenti...

#17) Doris Rapp, M.D., "Is This Your Child ? Discovering and Treating Unrecognized Allergies", Page 169, Quill, William, Morrow, NY, 1991

18) PURE FACTS Newsletter of the Feingold Association of the U.S., Europe and Food Dyes, Nov.2010, www.feingold.org

19) PURE FACTS Newsletter of the Feingold Association of the U.S., Food Dyes Pose a "Rainbow of Risks", July/Aug 2010. www.feingold.org

20) PURE FACTS Newsletter of the Feingold Association of the U.S., New Information on "Why Your Child is Hyperactive", Sept.2010, www.feingold.org

21) F.Batmanghelidj,M.D., "Your Body's Many Cries for Water", 2nd edition, Global Health Solutions, 1995, pg.120

22) Monday, July 13, 2009 by Paul Fassa,

www.naturalnews.com/026605_fluoride_fluorides_water.html

23) http://failsafediet.wordpress.com/about-food-chemical-intolerance/what-is-the-failsafe-diet/

CPSIA information can be obtained
at www.ICGtesting.com
Printed in the USA
LVOW01s0032010317

525683LV00004BA/381/P